A Love Story at the Seaside

All rights reserved.

Although I grew up in a small coastal town on the KwaZulu-Natal coast of South Africa very similar to where this story is set, and parts of this book reflect certain true incidents that have happened to people many years ago in this area of the world, this is a work of fiction.

Names, characters, places and incidents are used fictitiously. Any resemblance or similarities to actual places and events or persons, living or dead are entirely coincidental.

Ocean Sound, where this story takes place, is a fictitious name of a typical town along the KwaZulu-Natal South Coast, in South Africa.

No part of this publication may be reproduced, or transmitted in any form or by any means, electronic or otherwise, without prior written permission from the author.

First edition January, 2019

Copyright © 2019 Terry Atkinson

Contents

Chapter 1 5

Chapter 2 15

Chapter 3 20

Chapter 4 34

Chapter 5 44

Chapter 6 58

Chapter 7 67

Chapter 8 85

Chapter 9 90

Chapter 10 98

Chapter 11 105

Epilogue 120

A Love Story at the Seaside

Chapter 1

Robert caught another wave in the turbulent waters of the Indian Ocean and body-surfed it toward the shore. This was the first sunny day following several days of heavy rain in this small town called Ocean Sound. The Ocean Sound river had dumped its surplus load of muddy water into the cleansing salt of the ocean and Robert, along with 2 of his life-saving buddies, Peter and Mark, was enjoying the last few minutes after ending their training period.

Suddenly, Peter, who was further out, shouted "Swim for the beach – fast!"

Robert knew that could only mean one thing. He kicked furiously and stretched out his arms, using the force of the wave to flow his body as fast as he could toward the beach. Too late, just as he reached the shallow water and put out his leg to run, he felt the huge force of the shark as it grabbed his leg and shook his body up and out of the water, only to drag him back down into the warm Indian Ocean. Robert took what he thought was his last breath as the shark pulled him down while the waves crashed higher and higher above him.

Within seconds, the shark released his grip and was gone. The next wave washed Robert onto the beach where he pushed himself backwards away from the water's edge. He looked down on the blood-drenched leg, which was full of grainy beach sand. In total disbelief, Robert had one thought. *I thought that was my last breath, but I'm alive!*

Suddenly, he felt something tugging under his arms and pulling him back further onto the beach. "Call Bobby! Call Bobby!"

He realized that it was his life-saving team-mate, Peter, asking Mark to call their coach – who had already retired to the hut on the beach after their practice session for the upcoming surf lifesaving competition.

Bobby arrived on the scene within less than a minute, armed with the shark-attack kit containing a first-aid trauma kit and blood plasma. He immediately assessed the situation and contained the excessive bleeding with a tourniquet just above Robert's right knee.

"Put pressure on the artery," he said to Peter, as he wound a tight bandage around Robert's lower right leg. There was no time now to worry about all the sand that was mangled into the blood and tissue of the leg. Bobby right now, needed to save Robert's life and he was well aware that the nearest hospital was a 30 km drive away from this seaside village.

"Call Doctor Venter, then call the ambulance and traffic police. We'll need to get him to hospital as soon as he's stable. And get 2 of the boys in the hut to hook up and get us a fresh supply of plasma."

Mark hurriedly followed the coach's instructions, while Peter and Bobby competently stabilized one of their best life-savers, who was now in need of his own life being saved.

"Sophie – please let Sophie know," he managed to whisper through the haze of semi-consciousness that had overcome him since he had been lying on the beach, no longer having to fight this fight alone.

"Sure, Rob, we'll let her know. And your mom and dad. Just keep your energy, buddy," said Bobby reassuringly.

The next thing he knew, Doctor Venter was on the scene. The doctor gave Robert a shot of pentothal to anaesthetize and calm him down; and swiftly gave orders for the life-saver to be moved on the stretcher across the beach and to where the ambulance was parked. Once in the ambulance, he was further stabilized with the fresh supply of plasma being administered, thanks to his life-saving team-mates, and the driver was instructed to drive slowly to the closest hospital at that time, which was in Durban, almost 30 km north of Ocean Sound. Traffic had been cleared thanks to Mark's call to the traffic police and Robert was safely transported to the closest hospital in Durban.

~~~

"Hi honey," he heard the melodious tones of Sophie's voice as he battled to fight his way free of the blanket of anaesthetic which had numbed his awareness. Upon arrival at the hospital, 2 specialist surgeons had examined the damage done to his leg and reached a joint decision that, due to the extent and severity of the injury, it was not possible to save his lower leg. Robert had undergone a surgical amputation of his right leg just below the knee.

"Sophie," he smiled weakly as he gazed through the haze around his consciousness, up into those huge blue eyes he knew so well. Robert and Sophie had been dating steadily since high school and were known as Ocean Sound's sporting glamour couple. Sophie, a brilliant swimmer and diver in her own right, had a lot in common with Robert, who was a voluntary life-saver at Ocean Sound beach Surf Lifesaving Club and also represented his province as a diver. Sports and fitness had brought them together as a couple and they were admired by most locals for being quite an extraordinary couple with many sporting achievements already under their belts.

Robert saw the tears welling up in Sophie's eyes as she looked at her beloved Robert lying incapacitated in the hospital bed. No-one had told him that he'd lost his leg as a result of the shark attack. She didn't know what to say to him.

"It's going to be alright, Sophie. I survived! That's the important thing. I survived." He smiled up at her and lifted his hands to gently pull her face down towards his.

"Yes, that's right Rob," she said, sobbing quietly as he kissed her tears away from her eyes and cheeks.

"We're all gonna be OK," whispered Robert.

"Mom, Dad!" said Robert, suddenly becoming aware that his

parents, Martha and John, were standing behind Sophie.

"Sorry about this!" he grinned up at them. But the grin didn't last long. Why was everyone looking so upset and sad? He'd survived, hadn't he?

He should probably have known that it was not such a good idea to spend too long in the water that evening. The lagoon had been brown and general public swimming was banned on the beach that day. Ocean Sound's shark nets and drumlines could not be serviced during the bad weather conditions and were prone to lifting or damage. Thus, general swimming was never allowed after heavy rains, to protect the holiday makers and residents of this beautiful seaside town.

But due to the imminent surf lifesaving competition, Robert and his team had to make up for lost training time. They had agreed with their coach, to have a short training session that late afternoon. Now, here he lay in a hospital bed feeling the pain creeping into his leg as the drugs wore off.

"Hey guys, I'm alive! That shark didn't get the better of me," he said, trying to cheer everyone up.

"Robert, my boy, we need to tell you something." Robert looked up at his idol – his ruddy-complexioned, strong and athletic dad. Robert's dad was his hero. He always tried to follow his dad's example of kindness, manners and strength. His sister, Cindy, was working away in Cape Town so it was just his parents and his girlfriend, Sophie, who had come to see him today.

"What is it, dad?" asked Robert tremulously, feeling a sense of doom come into the hospital room.

"Robert," – said John, his voice quavering as Martha stood close and took his hand – "Robert, my boy, they had to cut your leg off."

Robert stared up at the trio of visitors and couldn't quite absorb what had been said. The images of their three concerned faces faded out as he tried to focus. The anaesthetic was still working out of his system.

"Just rest, Robbie. This is all too much right now. Please, just rest." His mom started sobbing as she stroked his hair back and plumped up the pillow. That was so typical of Mom. She would always handle her upsets by busying herself with something that would be good for somebody else.

Robert's heart sank. He sensed that his happy little family was never going to be the same again. He had lost a limb. But that was not all he was about to lose.

Chapter 2

"Hi Sophie," said Robert as he lurched unsteadily on his crutches, his right leg stump covered under the knee with a bright red stocking.

"Oh, my gosh, Robert, you're already up and on the move!"

Robert tried to ignore the look of shock and pain in his beloved Sophie's eyes. She tried not to look down at what was once his perfectly formed, strong, healthy, muscly leg. He was no longer physically the man that she had fallen for in the 11th grade. This was a rough moment for them both and they tried to make light of it.

"Let's see if I can get this body down to the coffee shop in the left wing."

Sophie walked slowly next to Robert as he struggled to manoeuvre his new crutches, heaving his one good leg along the cold floor. She smelled the antiseptic stink of all the cleaning fluids and felt sick to her stomach. *How could this have happened to us? Our lives were perfect. We were Ocean Sound's glamour couple,* she thought miserably to herself, trying not to show Robert what thoughts and feelings were swirling in a turmoil inside her.

"Sophie, I promise you, we can work this out," he said as he stirred his coffee slowly, having finally negotiated his long and arduous path to the coffee shop. "I can still dive, I can still swim. Hopefully by the time our lifesaving awards dance comes up, I'll be able to shuffle successfully on my artificial leg," he said, looking up at her pleadingly.

Sophie felt the wave of nausea come over her again. She was not used to seeing Robert appear anything but strong and confident. It broke her heart to see him so reduced in his manhood and life-force. He'd never had to plead with her about anything before. This was a new emotion for her to deal with.

"Robert, baby, let's take some time to adjust to all of this," she said, putting her hand on his. "We'll have to take this one step at a time."

He looked at those big, blue eyes and suddenly started laughing with abandon. All the pent-up stress of the past days seemed to release in a mad outburst of mirth, which didn't quite fit with the situation in which he found himself. The louder he laughed, the more perturbed Sophie became.

"Stop, Robert, it's not really funny! Look at us!'"

"Oh, Sophie," said Robert, helplessly clutching at his stomach as he went into another fit of hysteria. "One step at a time… don't you get it? I can't take one step at a time anymore. Do you get it?"

"That's not funny, Robert. That's just not funny."

Sophie went pale and knew she was going to throw up now. She dashed for the nearest loo and immediately lost her lunch she'd had prior to coming to visit Robert. She felt disgusted with herself and she felt awful for Robert. Life was simply not fair.

Robert leaned back into the plastic seat in the coffee shop. He tried so hard to see the brighter side of life. Still euphoric to some degree, that he hadn't capitulated fully in the ocean and lost his life, he had a strange sense of well-being despite the total tragedy that was happening to him regarding his physique. His mind whirled in a dizzy array of thoughts and "what ifs" and future possibilities. Seeing Sophie returning from the bathroom looking like a white ghost, Robert jolted in shock.

"Sophie, what's up? You look awful!" he exclaimed, extending his hand to help ease her down into the chair.

"Rob, it's all a bit much at the moment. This is such a shock and I'm not taking it very well," she sobbed as she let him hold her hand tightly. The sobbing became almost uncontrollable until Robert pushed her tea closer to her.

"Come on Sophie, we can face this together. We've always been a good team. I've lost my leg, not my heart. We can still laugh together, talk into the night and have fun together. I guess you'll beat me now when we run – but I can handle that."

Sophie looked up at the concern on Robert's face. In this moment she knew that this man was simply too good for her. She didn't deserve him. It was a moment of stark, cold truth and it sent a shiver down her spine.

"Sophie, put this on," said Robert, holding her cardigan out and helping her to put it around her shoulders.

Chapter 3

"One more lap, Robert. Let's work that leg and those hips!"

This is hell, thought Robert, sweating profusely as he went through his paces with Joe, his physiotherapist. Robert could not recall ever feeling this exhausted when he had trained in earlier times, running on the beach and swimming out against massive, crashing waves for the surf-lifesaving competitions.

After some time, Robert had been fitted with a prosthetic leg. He put a lot of effort into the intensive physiotherapy he received. Being the athlete that he was, he quickly got into the discipline of the daily exercises needed to strengthen the muscles in his upper leg. He knew this was the key to being able to walk as normally as possible on the artificial leg.

"OK that's good, Robert. Well done. We'll tackle this again in a couple of days. Soon we'll have you walking so that no-one would ever suspect it's not your leg."

Rob wrapped up his exercise session and shook Joe's hand. "Thanks for my torture session!" he grinned, doing his best, as usual, to see the lighter side of life. He knew that the harder Joe pushed him, and the harder he pushed himself, the better it was for him and those around him. He was used to pushing himself. He now had more personal reason to do so than before.

"Sure thing, Rob," said Joe. Joe was filled with admiration for the guts of this young man. His heart went out to Robert, who bravely faced the situation he was in by putting his attention on looking forward to his future, not looking back at the past and wallowing in self-pity. Robert accepted what had happened and put his focus on planning for and creating his future, which would now be different to his earlier sporting plans.

Joe had always had the deepest respect for the life-savers along the KwaZulu-Natal coastline. They risked their lives to save others, while most of the population were relaxing on the golden beaches and having a great time. Robert was one of the best lifesavers that Ocean Sound had ever had.

"I'll work out tomorrow in the pool, Joe, to work some different muscles. See you in two days for more of your treatment!" Robert grinned and waved as he made his way out of Joe's exercise room. Robert still swam as often as he could but for now, he avoided the ocean and swam laps in the indoor pool at the physio. He enjoyed the freedom from gravity more than ever before and it was in the water that he felt strong and able like he used to be.

His good friend from the lifesaving club, Peter, had finished his studies and decided to move up to Jo'burg to take a job offer there. Mark was still one of his best friends and although Robert couldn't join Mark anymore as a lifesaver, Robert invited him sometimes to train laps with him at the physio pool.

Soon, Robert was quite mobile without crutches. He was able to get up unaided and was walking better and better. When he returned to work, wearing his long pants, he merely walked with a slight limp – and to all intents and purposes, he was able to integrate into society and get back to his job in the marketing department of the largest sports store in the area, close to Ocean Sound. Rob resumed his university studies, which he was doing part-time through the main correspondence university in South Africa and he started to feel more normal again in terms of his work and studies.

~~~

These appearances did not match his personal life though, and Sophie continued to battle with the change that had occurred in both their lives. She was studying full-time at a fashion design college close to Durban. Her dream was to become one of the most innovative designers in the country for sporting and smart-casual wear. Sophie had dreams and goals that went with having a strong, able-bodied and handsome guy at her side, who would fit in with the fashion circles and the parties and society's expectations that came with such a career.

"Sophie, let's go out this Friday and start putting our lives back together," said Robert, trying to be cheery and act as if everything was as it used to be.

"Sure, Rob," said Sophie wanly, wondering how they could ever manage to re-create what they had before.

Sophie just knew she was going to dump Robert. And her heart ached as she also knew that it was not right. Sophie was a good person. But life had thrown her an unexpected curved ball. Nothing could have prepared her for this and she didn't know how to fix her attitude. The more she harboured these feelings of guilt, the more difficult it became to ask anyone for help. She didn't have the heart or the personal integrity and courage to raise the subject. She merely continued to put on an appearance that all was OK between her and Robert. She didn't want to put any more stress on this good man than he already had. But deep down, she knew that unless something fundamental changed in her, she was not going to pursue this relationship any further. She felt it a duty to keep up the act for now until Robert was settled again. That was the least she could do.

"How about a movie and then we can go to the pub over at the lagoon for a bite to eat afterwards," said Robert enthusiastically, happily anticipating a night out like the good old days.

"OK Rob, let's do that. I love sitting outside on the deck at that pub, watching the lights shining on the lagoon water.

"Yes, me too. It will be great to have some time together, Sophie, just to start planning again like we used to in the old days. We have lots to talk about because I've been so busy getting myself sorted out so I can live my life again."

Sophie's heart sank. *How much longer can I keep this up?* she wondered. She took a deep breath. "Of course, Rob. Let's meet at around 7 on Friday then, on the deck."

~~~

"Robert, this is really nice," said Sophie, twirling her straw in her cooldrink as they both sat on the outside deck of the pub, watching as the large, orange moon cast her light over the ripples in the lagoon. The pub was built right next to the water and the wooden deck reached out over the lagoon as it was poised on long wooden stilts which went down through the water into the earth below. At high tide, the water washed up close and splashed around the wooden stilts. Tonight though, it was low tide and sandy areas of the lagoon floor were exposed to view as the water flowed out toward the receding ocean.

In the distance, Sophie could see the lagoon spill out to join the infinity of droplets making up the Indian Ocean. Such a romantic place in the past, Sophie suddenly realized how she hated this lagoon now. It was the brown, murky water from this lagoon overflowing into the ocean, that had attracted that horrible shark which changed their lives forever.

A short distance away, in the soft moonlight, they could make out the white foam of the low tide waves of the ocean, backing off from the beach as they did at this time of the night. Sophie saw herself in the motion of those waves. She tried to go forward, then just as soon as she was moving in that direction, she backed off and retreated. Over and over, like the waves, Sophie could no longer find her forward direction with Robert. She felt trapped in an untenable position. *It's just his leg,* she thought, *how can I be so affected by it? I'm being selfish and ridiculous!*

But try as she did to reason the whole thing through, Sophie's emotions continued to get the better of her good sense and her basically kind heart. Sophie simply didn't know how to talk to Rob about what was going on with her internally.

"Yeah – romantic!" said Robert, holding her hand gently. "I've always loved coming to this spot with you, Sophie," he said, looking lovingly up at her face, which had a beautiful glow to it in the moonlight.

Sophie felt as if her heart would break in half right there. Here was this wonderful person who loved her and wanted to be with her. But some kind of selfish streak had overcome Sophie since the accident and no matter how hard she tried to pretend everything could go on as normal, she simply couldn't love Robert the same way anymore.

"Me too, Rob," said Sophie tremulously. "Listen, Rob," I just don't think that we can keep doing this," she blurted out.

"What's wrong, Sophie? I don't understand."

"Rob, I don't understand either. I don't understand myself, I don't know what's happened to me since the accident. I hate to have this discussion on such a romantic evening, Rob, but I simply can't go on with us. I just can't do it."

Robert looked at his girlfriend in utter disbelief. "Sophie, I thought we were getting our lives back together. I've recovered really well and I can walk and even jog sort of, and I can still swim. At least we can love each other and come out on dates like this.

When I was whirling around in that water feeling the warmth of my own blood, and when I was getting helped on the beach – I could only think of staying alive for you, Sophie. We have a future stretching out in front of us. Stretching out the way the ocean out there just keeps going on to the horizon and beyond. It's our future, Sophie – we can create it together. We can do this. Can't we leave the past behind?"

Sophie broke down into uncontrollable grief as she saw what her actions were doing to Robert. She felt like the worst person on earth. *I have to get this over and done with,* she thought.

"Robert, I think you will love me for being honest in the long run. I'm a bad person, Robert. I just can't carry on this relationship. We were together as 2 sporting, able-bodied people. This wasn't part of the deal. The last thing on earth that I want to do is add to your pain, Robert, but I can't pretend anymore that everything is fine. It might be fine with you, Robert. But it's simply not fine with me and I've tried everything I possibly can to make it right. But it isn't. You can call me the biggest bitch in the town, but I'm going to leave you, Robert. And you will do better with a kinder person than me. I don't deserve your love. You are a much better human being than me."

Robert stared aghast at his beautiful Sophie. He knew things had been tense between them since the accident, but this was a completely unexpected turn of events. He felt as if he'd been shot.

"Hey Sophie," said Robert gently, as he stroked her hair away from her pale face. He looked at this person who had once been his vibrant, sporty girl. He felt terrible at how much she had changed and gone downhill since his traumatic incident. Robert realized that he had new goals and dreams and things to strive for. Sophie had lost her joint goals with him.

Sophie couldn't bear this kindness after her cruel outburst. It was crazy. She wished that he would get mad at her. That's what she deserved. "It's just not working out between us since the accident, Robert. You know it and I know it. We need to go our separate ways."

Robert looked down, overcome with emotional agony. He felt a huge lump in his throat that wouldn't budge and he was unable to speak. When he finally managed to look up again, he saw the tears streaming quietly down Sophie's thin face.

"I didn't want this for us, Rob. We had it all on track. Our world was perfect. We were "Ocean Sound's couple". We can't ever get that back. And I can't do anything to change what has happened. Please take me home now, Robert," whispered Sophie. "I can't bear to be here with you anymore and hurt you more than I have."

Chapter 4

"Emma, darling, we are going to have to move," said her dear mom as she sat on her bed just before bedtime.

"I know, Mom," said Emma. They both understood why and it didn't need to be discussed further. It was time for Emma and her mom, Susan, to move on to a different place and start a new life away from memories.

"I've applied for that promotion – to run the branch office on the coast down in KwaZulu-Natal. I'm hearing tomorrow," said Susan, as she affectionately tucked a few loose strands of dark-brown hair away from Emma's soft, beautiful face. She noticed the tired look in her daughter's eyes. They needed to get away from this place which had once been so happy and full of laughter and life. Change was a great healer, and they both needed healing.

Susan, Emma's mom, was very hard-working. She managed to keep everything together with no man at her side to help with financial support. Life had been very tough for her and her only daughter, Emma, for the past 2 years. But Susan had worked her way up in her job and with careful planning, she'd kept up with all the bills and managed to get Emma through her schooling.

Now, a wonderful opportunity arose in the not very large town of Ocean Sound, right on the coastline. Properties were cheaper out there than moving closer to Jo'burg to chase more money, so expenses would be easier for Susan.

Emma smiled. *Good for you, Mom. I'm going to get that transfer now,* she thought happily. She had been waiting for this moment that they both so badly needed. Emma worked in a bank in Delmas, a farming town about 70km east of the big city of Johannesburg, economic hub of South Africa. Emma was born and raised in Delmas and only knew small town life. There were plenty of jobs in the other branches around the country and she had already told her boss that she might be looking for a transfer soon. For her and Mom, it was time to move away from the home that had given them such joy in earlier years and such heartache more recently. It was not only time to move away, it was time to open up a new chapter in their lives.

Within a week of her mom getting the promotion to run the branch of *Bob's Bed and Bathroom* store in Ocean Sound, Emma's transfer was also approved. For the next month while they worked their notice period, during weekends and after hours, they vigorously set about packing up their small house and getting ready for the move to a whole new zone. Ocean Sound was about 600 km from Delmas. They were going to be going far away from the town where Emma had grown up, gone to school and got her first job. *Time for a big change. Let's hope the nightmares will go away now,* thought Emma.

With the promise of some happiness and a future, the two women set off on their journey to the sea.

~~~

Emma walked into her new job with some apprehension. This was her first day at work since she and her mother had moved to Ocean Sound. Her new boss, Dave, showed her into her working space which was pretty similar to the bank where she had worked in Delmas. It was just quite a bit bigger.

"Hi guys, please welcome Emma. She's just arrived in town from the Delmas branch up in Mpumalanga. Small town like ours but she had a lot of dealings with our head office in Jo'burg. She'll need your help to get up and running in our little Ocean Sound branch but I'm sure we can all learn a thing or two from her and vice versa."

And so, here was Emma, walking into a group of staff who had mainly grown up in this small town and grown into jobs in the local bank branch. These people were used to hearing the sound of the ocean from the moment they woke up to the time they put their heads on the pillow to sleep. Emma had seen the ocean twice in her life prior to this move. She was the new girl and the stranger. Despite her excitement at starting out afresh, she was shy at the best of times, and this was not easy for her.

The noisy Monday morning chatter in the open-plan office came to an abrupt halt as Emma entered the space. A few of the guys drew in their breath suddenly at the sight of this beautiful, tall girl. Her cheeks flushed a healthy pink against her perfect, blemish-free skin and despite being an academic, rather than the sporty type, Emma was naturally fit and slim. She had grown up in a rural area where you had to walk or run bigger distances as a child to get to any place if you didn't have anyone to drive you there. When she wasn't studying, she would spend time outdoors, running around and climbing trees and she was not used to most modern conveniences. Their home never did have a TV set. There was just too much to do.

One could say that Emma was a natural beauty. And what made her even more beautiful, was that she had no clue that this was the appearance she put out there for others. She tended to be more focussed on her books and studying hard so that she could make it in this world economically. Since she lost her father while still at high school, she became very concerned about Mom having to carry the financial load and vowed to study hard and be successful so that she could bring her fair share to the household. Emma didn't really feel part of the usual crowd of kids going out partying on a Saturday night. She was an only child, a good student and she enjoyed her own company.

    Emma had seldom left Delmas to go into the big city, unless she had training for work or a meeting at head office. She valued the simple things in life – the things that mattered most to her – her love for her family and her appreciation of true friends who cared about her. Emma also enjoyed the outdoors and knew from an early age that a walk in the park cost nothing in hard cash, but gave back so much value to her spiritually. She had wanted to help her mom out as soon as she could land a good job. Mom had suffered enough and had made many sacrifices to keep the home fires burning. And Emma said many times to herself how she was going to return the help one day.

"Hi everyone," said Emma tentatively. "I hope I can do well here in your branch. I'm really happy to be here, right next to the ocean!"

"Hi Emma, I'm Jenna. I've been appointed to be your 'buddy' during your first week and will show you around here. Let's start with the coffee machine!" said Jenna sweetly. Dave couldn't have chosen a nicer person to help Emma to get used to her new environment. Jenna had been at the branch for a year since graduating from high school and was one of the youngest staff members at the bank.

"Thanks Jenna," said Emma, smiling brightly at this sweet and pretty girl. She started to feel more relaxed and hoped her mom was having an easy time at her new job too.

"Hey Emma, a few of us go walking on the promenade sometimes on a Saturday if you want to join us? You can meet my brother, Mark and another good friend of his, Robert. They are volunteer life-savers who work on the beach during their spare time. That way you can get to meet more people in the town.

We might as well do it now during the quiet season, because once all the holiday-makers from Jo'burg come down to invade our ocean, there won't be space to breathe out there," she said with a mischievous grin. Jenna was referring to the mass invasion of holiday-makers who came in their droves from landlocked Jo'burg and surroundings near Emma's home town every summer to swamp the beaches of this quiet little seaside town.

"Sure Jenna, that would be nice. Thank you for inviting me." Emma started to feel that she might be able to experience happiness again. It was the first time she'd felt that way since the tragedy that she and her mom had gone through, preceding their departure from Delmas.

Chapter 5

"Meet Emma, Rob!" said Mark with a wink. "She's new in town. And works in the same bank as my sister."

Robert looked at this gorgeous, dark-haired beauty as Mark touched her affectionately on her arm.

"I'm showing her around the place because she's a bit shy and Jenna asked me to help out. We thought to go for a walk on the promenade later today if you want to join us?"

"Hi Robert," said Emma, holding out her hand to shake Rob's. "Jenna and Mark have told me about you and what a great sportsman you are!"

Robert winced a little inwardly. He wondered how much had been told. Robert only wore long pants these days, and managed to walk fairly well with only a hint of a limp. He didn't go out there advertising the fact that he had half a leg missing.

"I'd love it if you could join me, Jenna and Mark later. I don't have many friends here yet, and it will be nice to go out together."

Wow, Mark! You've met a wonderful woman, thought Robert as he looked at her kind eyes, smiling back at him. He wondered if Mark had eyes for her, or if he was simply helping Jenna out with her work buddy. *Wouldn't be a bad choice if you went for her, Mark,* thought Robert, hoping that his friend might finally find a girl that he could feel comfortable with.

"I'd love to join you guys! After the walk, maybe we can go down to the lagoon pub and grill. They should be showing the rugby there on the big screen."

"Great idea!" said Mark enthusiastically. He was happy that Robert was getting back to his social life again after his horrible accident.

"Hi Sophie!" said Mark, seeing the tall, blond, well-tanned woman walking towards them on the prom. She didn't answer at first, then as she drew closer, she removed the wireless headphone that she had perched in her ear – she was listening to her favourite music she liked to walk to.

"Hi guys," the perfect, white teeth flashed as she managed a friendly grin, including Robert in her greeting. "Who's the new girl?"

"Sophie, this is Emma – she's new in town.

"Hi Sophie, nice to meet you," said Emma, blushing with shyness. *This has to be one of the most beautiful women I've ever seen! The guys must all be crazy about her,* she thought quietly to herself. Emma felt a little inadequate around such a confident and clearly athletic and fit girl. She felt so out of place here, with these physically well-built people who were used to swimming and working out. Emma felt very pale against their tanned skins.

"Hi! So, you've met some of the guys, then," said Sophie. "They'll show you around and give you a good time. Just make sure they behave!" she said with a little giggle as she hurriedly went ahead with her walk. She couldn't stand the pain of seeing Robert there, putting on this show of walking normally and wearing long pants when everyone else was in shorts. *I have to get away from here,* she thought as she put the headphone back in her ear.

~~~

"Hi guys!" Fiona smiled as she saw some of her favourite customers coming into the grill-house for a good time tonight. She liked Mark and Robert because they were professional sportsmen and they didn't drink more than they should on a night out - unlike some of the rowdier customers she sometimes had to handle during holiday season.

"You want to sit over here so you have a good view of the big screen? Rugby match starts in about half an hour, I think," she said, bustling around and ensuring there were enough chairs at her proposed table.

"Sure, Fiona, that would be great! Are you serving us tonight? Robert smiled happily as he pulled out a chair for Emma to his left and Jenna to his right. "You sit next to Emma on the other side, Mark. Then she has us two men to take care of her in case the drinkers get out of hand."

Mark winked at Robert. They both knew that during quiet season this little pub seldom got totally crazy like it could do in Durban, the closest city. Too many people knew each other in this town, and had to face up to unimpressed looks on a Monday morning at work if they overdid things. Mostly, it was decent folk who frequented 'Oswald's Pub and Grill'. They enjoyed hanging out with each other at the end of the week and it was the most fun place to watch a big rugby match, as there was a great atmosphere and spirit of friendship in the wooden logged pub on the lagoon. Additionally, they served the most delicious steaks and pizzas for miles around.

"OK guys, thank you!" said Emma gratefully. She was looking forward to watching the match along with her new friends and felt at ease with this group. She knew that Mom was safely at home and enjoying a quiet night with her book and this was her first chance since moving here, to let her hair down a bit and relax.

"Fiona, this is Emma. She's from up north – near Jo'burg. But she's also from a small town and she's moved here now. You'd better take her drink order as you know what the rest of us usually have," said Mark happily.

"Hey Emma, nice to meet you. Hope they're treating you nicely and helping you to find out where all the nice places are around here. And I sure hope this is the first restaurant they brought you to, because of course, we are the best at 'Oswald's'!" grinned Fiona. "So, what's it going to be love, a draught of beer with the boys?"

"Oh, I'll have a lime and soda thanks, Fiona. That goes down well in this heat!"

"Sure honey, I'll be right back with the first round for everyone."

Within no time, the countdown came for the big rugby match. Everyone was contentedly settled with their drinks and the dinner orders had gone through to the busy kitchen. The grill-house was getting fuller and fuller and Emma now realized why they'd met here much earlier than the start of the match. It was, after all, a Saturday night and the people of Ocean Sound were having a good time after their busy week at work.

"There they go!" yelled Robert, excitedly watching the players come out on the pitch to sing their National Anthems. Hope we give the Aussies a good hiding!"

From this point on, the entire pub was riveted to the screen, focussing on the very close and exciting match. At half-time, they ate their delicious food and chattered eagerly about the game and how it was likely to turn out.

Almost forty minutes later, it was an even score and the tension was mounting. "It's a foul! We've got a penalty!" roared Rob – the most vociferous of all the spectators. He really loved his rugby, and if he hadn't shown so much talent for swimming and diving, he might have played professionally. The room went quiet as everyone waited for the player to kick. They all seemed to be holding their breath. Then the flags went up at the posts and the whistle blew. "It's through! He got it through! We've won!"

A loud roar of applause and hugging and clinking of glasses rushed through the happy bunch of people enjoying to see their country win against the formidable *Wallabies,* the very strong Australian rugby team. It was a little too close for comfort, but a win is a win!

Robert turned to Emma and gave her a huge, bear-like hug. "You brought us luck, Emma! That's the first time we've won in a long time! You can come and watch rugby with us anytime!"

"Ah thanks, Robert! I'm sure it had absolutely nothing to do with me, but I'd love to do this again. It's been such fun!"

She looked up at him with sparkling eyes, her dark hair glistening in the bright lights of the restaurant. Suddenly, she was struck with how handsome Robert was. She had never really noticed that before. The first thing she'd been aware of was what a kind and decent guy he was. And it didn't seem fair to her that he'd had such a sad thing happen to stop him in his sporting career. She also knew from Jenna that Robert and Sophie had broken up since the accident. That seemed to be so unfortunate to Emma's mind.

"Sure, Emma, any time! You're always welcome in our group. If you're Jenna's friend, you're our friend." He put his arm on Emma's and gave it a warm, friendly squeeze.

Emma blushed, and hoped that he wouldn't notice. She felt a pang of sadness at the attention she was getting from such a nice man. And to top it all, suddenly she noticed Sophie, out of the corner of her eye, glancing her way. Sophie was sitting with a bunch of her sporting friends and fellow-students from her fashion design college. They were in their own group. Emma became very uncomfortable. "Robert, it's been a lovely night! I think I should be leaving now. I came with Mark and Jenna, but it's early enough for me to walk home – I live not too far from the beach in the apartments up the road."

"Oh, it's fine, Emma, I'll walk you home," said Robert quickly.

"No, it's totally OK Rob, Mom is up and I'll be perfectly safe." She hurriedly gathered her handbag and gave some cash to Jenna towards their joint bill.

"Emma, please stay a bit longer," said Jenna as she saw that Emma was about to leave. "I don't want to be the only girl here. Come with me quickly to the bathroom please, even if you need to go home afterwards."

"OK Jenna," said Emma, feeling for Jenna being left with the guys in this noisy place. Her group had not had much alcohol. In fact, both Mark and Robert had stopped after their first beer. But others were getting noisier and noisier the more they drank and it wasn't such a nice place to be anymore. She stepped down off her bar stool and went off with Jenna to the bathroom.

"Emma, please just stay on a little while – we usually end off with a coffee and then we'll be out of here. And Mark and I will drive you home. You're new in this town and you don't know the place at night. We can't have you walking home on your own. And I understand if you don't want to go alone with Robert."

"Jenna, Sophie's here – did you see her? I don't want to get involved with anyone's ex. I actually am not interested in getting involved with anyone right now," said Emma, her eyes filling with tears.

"Em, come and wash your face a little bit. You'll feel better. Let's just go back to the guys and order some coffees, then we'll take you home. It's been such a lovely, fun night. Let's not spoil it now. We like this place to watch the rugby and get together on the weekends. But none of us like it when it gets too late and some of the people get too drunk. We don't want you to feel bad on your first night out with us."

"Alright, you've convinced me. But you sit next to Robert then, and I'll sit next to you."

The girls made their way back to the table and ordered coffees for everyone. Within a short time, the group got ready to leave.

"Thanks Fiona, for another great night at 'Oswald's'! We had a wonderful time!"

"Sure guys! See you again soon!"

They said their goodbyes to Robert in the parking lot near to his car. Emma, feeling a bit strange still, but not wanting to hurt Robert's feelings, gave him a hug goodnight and he kissed her quickly on the cheek. He did the same with Jenna and Emma relaxed a little.

"Bye, Rob!" they waved to him as he climbed a little awkwardly into his modified automatic car to drive home to his cottage which he lived in on his parents' property.

"See you next Saturday for our walk on the prom!" he said through the open window, as he drove off into the night.

"Thanks guys, for running me home. And thanks for a beautiful night out on the town – my new town!" said Emma as she hugged Mark and Jenna goodbye. Mark seemed taller when she stood close to him and she was aware of how strong his body felt as she hugged him. He was a really nice man.

Emma wondered why he didn't have a girlfriend. Some lucky girl was missing out.

Chapter 6

"Thanks for meeting me, Emma," said Sophie anxiously. She stood up a little hesitantly to greet Emma, who looked more stunning than ever as she approached the little round table which had a view directly onto the beach and the ocean. *How does she do it? She doesn't diet, she doesn't work out or anything,* thought Sophie jealously.

It was a few weeks after their first meeting on the promenade. Sophie and Emma had met again in the town a couple of times since then. It was also not lost on Sophie that on the night they all watched rugby at 'Oswald's Pub and Grill', Robert could hardly take his eyes off Emma, even though she had come to the pub with Mark and Jenna and not with Robert.

"No problem, Sophie, it sounded quite urgent, so of course I'm happy to meet with you. What's up?" smiled Emma so sweetly, it went through Sophie like a knife.

How can I be such a bitch? She thought, as she motioned to Emma to take a seat.

"Emma, there's something I have to tell you because it's eating me up inside."

Emma looked quietly at Sophie, waiting for her to speak further. She was totally surprised in the first place that Sophie had wanted to meet with her. Sophie was one of the "in" girls in the town and didn't seem to want to mix much with Emma at all. In fact, Emma felt a little intimidated by Sophie's confidence which came from her sports and her popularity. She wondered what on earth could be on her mind.

"Go ahead, Sophie, I'm willing to listen."

"Emma, I know that Robert is growing more and more fond of you. It's your right, if you want to date him. I am not good enough for him. But please, don't mess him around. Don't just date him because you feel sorry for him and use him until someone better comes along. Because if you do, I'll never forgive you."

Emma stared at Sophie for a long, uncomfortable pause. She was stunned by the communication, because dating Robert was the last thing on her mind. She then turned her gaze to the grey-blue ocean waves, crashing down onto the beach some metres from the window of the coffee shop. She shuddered inwardly, thinking briefly about Robert, and what he must have experienced during that horrific incident where he lost half his leg. She knew more about the incident now because Jenna had told her in private, simply out of care for Robert that he didn't get unnecessarily embarrassed. But Emma had not raised it directly with Robert. She felt that it was up to Robert if he wished to discuss it and they were frankly, not that close.

"I don't know what you're talking about, Sophie. What do you mean, he's growing fond of me? What has he said to you?"

Sophie's glittering blue eyes suddenly filled with big pools of tears. "You bitch!" she sneered, as she grabbed her handbag to leave.

"Sophie! That's not on!" Emma felt anger rising within her. This was not an emotion she liked and it was not one that she was accustomed to feeling. But something was very wrong here and she was not going to let this jealous girl stand up and walk out on her, especially after such an invalid accusation. Besides, Sophie was the one who had invited her for coffee so she could jolly well stay and have the meeting.

Sophie almost crumpled under Emma's iron grip as she settled back into her chair.

"What is really going on, Sophie? I hardly know you. You know that I'm not after Robert – I've only recently met him. So, what's *really* going on?" Emma's voice had softened now, as she saw that this super-fit, glamour girl suddenly looked like a little lost creature with no place to go. Streaks of mascara started to line her face as she groped furiously in her bag for a Kleenex. Sophie tried desperately to summon some form of dignity and quieten her sobbing as Emma quietly sat, waiting for an answer to her question.

"He loved me, and only me. Our lives were perfect. We were inseparable and everyone knew that I was his girl. Then that accident changed everything," she almost whispered, as her sobbing subsided.

"Why did it have to change things, Sophie? He's the same man. He's missing part of a limb. But why would that have to change your relationship?"

"You don't understand, do you?" said Sophie, becoming bitter and combative again.

"Do you know anything about me, Sophie? How could you judge whether I understand or not?"

Sophie suddenly looked at Emma with new eyes. This girl was no pushover. She stood her ground and didn't just capitulate to Sophie's confidence the way other weaker people did. She found herself liking Emma despite the situation she felt she was in.

"OK, you're right. So how would you know what it feels like to have a boyfriend who was the most handsome guy in the town, the best in all the sports and above all, my one and only love, who then gets half his leg bitten off while he's doing his favourite sport?"

"Sophie, I can't say I know what that feels like. But at least you still have Robert around. If you cut off half your hair, does he have to dump you? If you file your finger nails and lose those parts of your body, or lost a tooth - aren't you still there afterwards? I know you can't really compare that to losing a limb, Sophie – but it's just to make the point. Robert, the being, is still there. He can still breathe, communicate and love! Sophie, it's not all about the looks, the body parts, the muscles. It's about the human being that you love."

Sophie looked at Emma in shock. Her words were like daggers into her heart. She knew that Emma was right. She just hadn't had the guts to face this truth up until now, and here was this new girl in town teaching her a lesson – but in the nicest possible way. "Emma, how can you be so wise? I know you're right. I just hate myself for not being able to love him anymore. You deserve him more than I do. You should start dating him if you want to – he does like you."

Emma looked at Sophie and smiled.

"Sophie, if you really love him, you will find that you are able to love him just as he is, for who he is. You should simply look at that and decide if you really love *him*, or his looks. Because you will find the answer there to hating yourself. You don't need to do that to yourself or to Robert. Look at what you really love about Robert and re-kindle that. Look at all the good times you had together, your favourite moments when you laughed together. Was it the body you loved? Or was it Robert, the person, whom you loved? If it's true love, Sophie, you'll be able to love him just as you did."

Sophie listened attentively. She saw the sense in what Emma was putting out there for her to look at. "Emma, you have really helped me today, and I had intended something else entirely for this meeting. Thank you for having the courage to stand up to my nonsense. I won't forget what you've done for me today. I'm going to try what you suggest. I might just need another coffee date in a while to update you on how it goes – and I promise not to attack you."

"That would be lovely, Sophie. I'm glad that I could help," smiled Emma, relieved that this girl was no longer so upset and full of blame.

"Emma, I don't know what planet you come from, but they taught you some really good sense there," said Sophie, putting her hand in a friendly gesture on Emma's arm. "Wherever you learned your wisdom, they did a good job of teaching you."

If only you knew, Sophie. If only you knew, thought Emma, not able to confide in this volatile girl, what had really happened that led to her and her mother coming to this town.

Chapter 7

Emma sat quietly in her lonely lounge. Mom was working late as usual and the supper that she had prepared would need to be heated up when Mom got home. Emma tried to get into the novel she was reading, to keep her mind occupied. She hated too much time to think about things. That's when the horrible memories came back to her. Nobody in this new town knew why she and her mom had arrived here to restart their lives.

Giving up on the novel, she tossed the book down and got up to put on some music. Anything to take her attention off the things she tried so hard not to think about, every day of her life since the tragedy.

Suddenly, her phone rang. "Emma, it's Robert." Emma's world whirled in that instant. She thought about the conversation with Sophie. It never occurred to her that Sophie could, in fact, be right. She just thought Sophie was jealous and bitter.

"Hi Robert," the words came out nervously, as she didn't know what to expect.

"Emma, I need your help with something. Are you able to meet me tomorrow morning down at the pool end of the promenade? I'd like to meet you there early before the usual beach-lovers arrive. I'm free from 8.30 a.m."

Although this request puzzled her a little, Emma thought it would be a good opportunity to straighten things out with Robert and let him know what had been going on with Sophie. She would ask him to perhaps talk to Sophie about it so that she didn't get falsely accused again of trying to steal Sophie's old boyfriend.

"Sure, Robert. I'll see you tomorrow at 8.30 a.m." said Emma firmly.

Fortunately, Emma and her mom lived in a little apartment within walking distance to the promenade and the beach. So, she'd be able to get there tomorrow without having to ask Mom if she could use the car that they shared.

Happy to have something else to think about, Emma started to get out the dinner plates. Mom should be arriving home soon. Just then, she heard the rattling of the key in the door as her beloved mother finally came in so that they could enjoy a dinner together.

"I'm meeting up with Robert tomorrow, Mom, he wanted some help with something."

"What a sweet boy," said Susan, looking tenderly at her only child. She so wished that Emma would get more happiness in her life. She had had to endure so much and it was time for Emma to have some good fortune. She was wise beyond her years, due to what she'd been through, and Susan would never have wished for her daughter to have grown up so quickly. But life wasn't always kind or fair and Emma had undergone more than her fair share of cruel circumstances. Susan thought that they would both be happier at this small, seaside town and she was glad to see her daughter starting to fit in with some of her friends.

~~~

"Hiya Emma!" Robert was waving vigorously from near the tidal pool. Emma was startled to see that Robert was sitting on the rock near the pool without his prosthetic leg. He had swimming trunks on – with a bright, green and blue pattern. At the end of his right stump, he had the same patterned material neatly covering the stump and reaching over the knee. Robert looked happy but slightly nervous. The beach area was practically deserted, apart from a few early-morning fishermen who had set up their positions on the outcrop of rocks a little way away.

"Hi Robert! What a beautiful day for a swim!" said Emma, anticipating Robert's next move.

"Yes! I wanted to see how I do with my diving, having to hop very cautiously to the end of the board," he said, winking a little mischievously at Emma.

"Emma, you are the only person around who never saw me dive at competition level when I had both my legs the same length. I wanted to do this on my own the first time, but then I thought I might need a little help and the best person I could think of that I could trust, was you. You have not judged me since the first time we met, and you aren't caught up in my past in this town. I just thought it would be nice if you were here."

"Gosh Robert, that's quite a choice you made! I have never really been a swimmer! I grew up in a little place that occasionally had water in the dam – in the summer months. But we just goofed around in that water! I can stretch out my hand from the side to help you out if needed! But I'm no life-saver if you land in trouble!"

"Oh, the swimming part is not the problem – it is just getting out to the end of the board and making sure I'm stable before I dive. You'll do just fine, Emma, if I need you."

Emma smiled softly. She felt happy today. It was a gorgeous, sunny day and the beach seemed to belong totally to them as it was not holiday season yet. During the quiet times, you could really enjoy a day out here in the fresh air, with the water crashing constantly in your ears and the seagulls soaring through the blue skies above. She was glad that her mom had decided to move here and for the first time in a very long while, Emma could see that she might be able to move on from the past and create a sunnier future here for herself. She admired this man, Robert. He had also had his share of hard luck and here he was, enthusiastically trying out his old skill and not letting the past hamper him.

"Okey dokes, Robert! Just take it easy and I'm right here!" said Emma, thankful that she was wearing shorts and a light shirt, in case she got wet during this exercise. Robert had not prepared her for this so she was not exactly "dressed" for the occasion with a bathing suit.

Robert used light, aluminium crutches to get up to the diving board and then handed them carefully to Emma before hauling himself up by the hand rails on each side of the steps up onto the board. Emma then watched in utter amazement, as he hopped gently on the slightly springy board - and then steadied himself at the end. He bent on his left leg and lifted up like a swallow into the air, and executed a simple, but beautiful dive, cleanly through the air and then straight down into the water, cutting through it like a kingfisher after his bait.

"Wow, you're really good!" said Emma excitedly from the side of the pool, as Robert came up for air, grinning like a Cheshire cat. "I had no idea!"

"Thanks, Em! That's a breakthrough moment for me! Excuse the pun. I wasn't sure how it was going to go, having to hop down that board and then dive cleanly into the water! It felt almost like the old times once I was in the air. What a win!!"

"Here you go," said Emma, extending her hand to help Robert clamber onto the side of the pool. "Let's see another one!"

"Sure! Since we're the only ones out here this morning, you'll get the first diving show from me since my recovery."

After a little while of Robert testing out what he could still do, despite the change in balance he was experiencing, he hauled himself up onto the side next to Emma and grinned. "That's enough for my first time out. I'm exhausted! Thanks for being here, Emma – it made it a lot easier for me to face up to this."

"I'm happy I could help, Robert. I didn't really do much!" Emma smiled happily and leaned back on the rock, enjoying the company of this amazing guy. They both sat for a while, taking in the mainly blue scenery. It was one of those really clear days, where the horizon of the ocean almost blended into the sky in the sunny haze. Emma loved the never-ceasing sound of the thundering roar of the waves, crashing over the rocks near the tidal pool, and then, their force spent, rolling tamely up onto the yellow, granular beach. She thought briefly of her little town where she grew up and then turned her attention to the present. She knew she and Mom had made the right move. They were missing nothing back there.

This was where they would build their new lives.

"Robert," said Emma quietly, "I want to talk to you about something."

"Shoot, Emma," said Robert, enjoying sitting here with this sweet girl. He had not been able to get Sophie out of his mind since they broke up and he still loved her despite everything. But it was nice to enjoy the company of this fresh, new girl in town.

"Robert, Sophie and I have met a few times for coffee. She's really mad at herself for what happened between you and her. I know it's none of my business, but I tried to help her. I know that deep down, she still loves you. But she's battling with what happened."

Robert's face tightened with emotion. Emma got nervous, sensing that she'd stepped on a very raw nerve. "Sorry, Robert, I don't mean to upset you. I just thought I should tell you. Because I think she would like to work things out but she has to come to terms with it in her own mind first. I don't really know how to help her more – but I wanted to let you know that we had been talking, because it doesn't seem right to do that behind your back."

"I'll always love Sophie, Emma. We were high school sweethearts and life seemed to be made for her and me to be together. But life doesn't always work out the way it seems. She doesn't want me the way I am, Emma. I know that. I have to come to terms with it and move on with my life. And she should do the same."

"OK Robert. I'm sorry I raised it. I know it's none of my business."

"Hey, it's alright, Emma. You are a sweet girl. I know you only mean well. Come – let's get out of here now – I've totally tired myself out. Could you bring over the crutches for me?"

Robert and Emma made their way slowly back to the promenade and headed for his car, which was parked in the parking lot a little way away. Robert navigated expertly with his crutches using the path along the area of hardened, wet sand closer to the tidal pool. It could get tricky in the softer, granular sand on the main beach. She helped him to load the crutches so that he could reach them from the back when he got home.

"Thanks again, Emma," said Robert, giving her a little kiss on the cheek. "Today was really the start of my new life."

"Glad I could be there for you, Robert." Emma was a little embarrassed by the peck on her cheek. She hoped that Sophie was nowhere in sight. She waved nervously as he reversed his automatic car out and turned toward the main road leading away from the beach.

Emma started to walk the short distance along the promenade back to the path through to her apartment. It was faster to walk than to go by car from this particular point. After a lovely morning enjoying the sea, sunshine and Robert's company, she now started to feel a little uneasy.

~~~

"Hi Emma!" Emma looked up to see Sophie waving from the bench along the prom. She drew in a quick breath, wondering if she'd seen her and

Robert at the pool. "I came out here to think a bit – it's such a beautiful day, isn't it?"

Emma smiled at Sophie. She looked happier today than the last time they had met. "Yes! It's not too hot and not to cool. I was just down at the pool – I met Robert there at his request," said Emma, blurting it out before she could stop herself. She was the new girl in town and she didn't want any untrue rumours to be spread about her.

Sophie's smile turned to a hard, accusing look which made Emma's stomach churn.

"It's not what you think, Sophie. Honest. We can call Robert here and he can tell you."

"What game are you playing, Emma, coming to this town to mess up our lives? Why don't you and your mother just pack your bags and go back to where you belong!"

"Sophie, please! I'm telling you, it's not what you think." Emma grabbed Sophie's arm and sat down firmly next to her. Once again, she was not going to allow the over-emotional Sophie to read things the wrong way. She held her ground and insisted on sitting down next to Sophie and calming her down.

By now, Sophie was crying and in a total state. People were starting to walk on the prom as the beachgoers began to come out after their weekend sleep-in.

"Come with me, Sophie – I live just around the corner. Let's go and talk somewhere private."

Emma gently coaxed Sophie to walk next to her and led the way up the path to her apartment. "Here, I always carry these around because the wind gets up my nose!" she said, as she fished a Kleenex out of her pocket and thrust it into Sophie's hand.

"Here we go – it's not a castle, but it's home to us, and walking distance to the beach!" said Emma, opening up their slightly tired-looking apartment door and showing Sophie to the second-hand couch in their modest lounge. She opened up the windows to let the sea breeze in and to get the soft roar of the ocean into her lounge. She loved this sound and felt it had a calming effect.

"Can I get you a coffee or a cool drink?" she said, bustling off to the kitchen which was open-plan, so she could continue the conversation with Sophie from in front of the fridge. "Mom's gone to work this morning, so it's just us."

"Just a glass of water, thanks," said Sophie, annoyed with herself for breaking down in front of Emma. She kept on mis-estimating this stranger from out of town. And it particularly annoyed her that whenever she wanted to get really mad at her, she could find no cause for it.

"Here you go, said Emma, bringing through 2 tall glasses of cold water from the fridge, and settling down in the wicker chair opposite the couch where Sophie was sitting, sniffing a bit and wiping her eyes with a fresh Kleenex.

"Robert asked me to join him this morning, Sophie. He did something really brave. I felt quite uncomfortable that he invited me to do that and I wished you had been around."

Emma proceeded to tell Sophie about her morning with Robert and his achievements on the diving board.

"That's the Robert I fell in love with, Emma. That's the kind of guy he is. He never gives up and he never accepts defeat."

Emma looked at the expression in Sophie's eyes. Still watery with emotion, Emma could see that Sophie really did still love Robert.

"This is totally ridiculous," she said suddenly. The two of you are in love! You should just work it out. You are so darn annoying, both of you!"

Sophie was totally startled at this outburst from Emma and stared at her in astonishment.

"I'm phoning Robert right now," said Emma, on a roll now, "and I'm calling him over here. You two have to talk to each other and straighten this all out. I can't stand it! And I'm not getting in the middle of it anymore!"

"How dare you, Emma! This is absolutely none of your business. You have no right meeting up with my boyfriend on your own and you have no right running our lives. You're a stranger in this town and you know nothing of our past."

Suddenly, Emma's phone rang.

"It's Robert," said Emma in a low voice. "Who's going to take this call? You or me?"

Chapter 8

A couple of weeks had passed by since Sophie finally got the courage to talk to Robert and meet with him to work things out one way or another. Thanks to Emma's pressure, they were at least able to communicate civilly with each other and be seen together again on social occasions. It was extremely difficult for both of them but they persevered. Life was still better having each other as friends than not seeing each other at all.

Emma did her best to put her head down at work and concentrate on doing the best she could at her job. She was growing to like this little town and wanted to ensure she had a career here and could continue on at the bank. She felt she had interfered enough now, in Sophie and Robert's affairs, and tried to keep out of their business.

Mark and Jenna had become her firm friends and quite often, they would meet when the rugby was showing at the pub and grill at the lagoon. They often also bumped into Sophie and

Robert there, and the group made social plans together. It seemed to suit Robert and Sophie to be part of the group, but not considered a romantic couple at this point. They both needed time.

"Hey Emma," said Sophie one day when they were sitting out on the wooden deck of the pub, waiting for their friends to join them. "Why don't you and Mark get together? I know you're not going to mess with my man – well, ex-man - but Mark is single. He's available. You two would make a great couple!"

Sophie was shocked to see the tears glisten in Emma's eyes as she made this friendly comment. She realized she'd touched a very sensitive nerve in the girl who seemed to always have nerves of steel, and held her space no matter what threats or challenges came her way.

"Hey, sorry, Emma – I didn't mean to upset you! You've never told me anything about you and your past, really. It was always all about me!"

"It's OK, Sophie. It's a long story and one that I'd rather forget about." Emma quickly brushed her arm across her face to wipe away the wetness as she saw Robert, Mark and Jenna coming through the door of the restaurant.

"Hey, there come the rest of the 'crew'. Let's have a good time and hope that the *Sharks* win!" said Sophie quickly. The official name of the rugby team in this region which bordered the ocean, had been a point of discomfort at times with Robert around. But they had all moved on now and everyone was used to the fact that Robert was back to being one of the boys, and not so sensitive anymore to allusions to his accident.

"Hi guys!" Robert entered ahead of the others with a big grin on his face. It's going to be a blast, all of us watching the rugby. Glad everyone could make it!" He touched Sophie gently on her shoulder and leaned over to kiss her briefly. They were still a little awkward and it pained the others to see that the once hand-in-glove couple had not yet been able to fully resolve the situation and get back together in the way that they had been. Robert then kissed

Emma on the cheek and settled in a spot between the two.

Mark pulled up an extra chair to make enough seats at their wooden table, and sat next to Emma on one side and his sister on the other. Within a few minutes, they'd all ordered their drinks and a few pizzas to share. It was going to be a fun night out. They were all wearing their *Sharks* T-shirts and hoped that they would defeat the *Lions* from Jo'burg. Luckily for Emma, she was happy to support the *Sharks* as she was from another province, and was not expected to back up the *Lions* from Jo'burg.

"This is home now," said Emma cheerily. "I'm a *Sharks* supporter through and through! Here's to a great match!" They clinked their glasses together and laughed happily as they looked forward to the match ahead and a good time all round amongst friends.

Chapter 9

"Sophie, do you remember you asked me once how I would know what it felt like to have a boyfriend who had suffered a physical trauma. I told you I wouldn't know what that felt like. Well, there is something more I want to mention on that."

The two girls were spending some time in Sophie's apartment on a Saturday morning. Later they'd be joining the others on the promenade and might even take a dip in the ocean after that, as it was very hot today.

"What is that, Em?" asked Sophie enquiringly. She hadn't tried to scratch more in the area of Emma's potential love-life after seeing how emotional she got when she had suggested Mark as a possible partner. She braced herself for what Emma was about to put on the table.

"Sophie, you have Robert. He lived through his ordeal. You can create a future with him if you just decide to. You must have laughed together and planned together. That didn't need both his legs to do that. I've already tried to get you to see that...to see that he's still the same guy as before the shark attack.

He might have some different emotions and memories, but it's still Robert, the Robert that you knew. You yourself told me that he was doing the same things now, when he asked me to watch him dive. He's the same person, taking up a challenge and overcoming it. His challenges are just a little different. But *he* is no different. His personality is the same. You are actually lucky that he didn't become bitter and twisted and start living a life of feeling sorry for himself."

Sophie listened attentively. She had learned the hard way, to hear Emma out when she had something important to say.

"Sophie, I'm not super religious, but I do know that we are not our bodies – that there's more to us than just the meat and bones that make up our bodies. We are spiritual beings and we use our bodies to enjoy life and go out and eat and swim and dance and stuff.

Our bodies are just vehicles that we inhabit as spiritual beings and we recognize each other by our bodies. We obviously want to have good-looking bodies, and dress them nicely and make them look pretty for others. But our bodies are not who we really are. They simply represent, physically, who we are. Robert is a spirit - a soul, inhabiting a body that has an imperfection. You are a spirit and you look after your body well and have a nice body to present to the world."

This was the first time that Emma had talked so deeply, in such a philosophical way. Sophie knew that Emma had a wise outlook on life and this was the furthest she'd ever expressed herself in exposing her personal viewpoints. She wondered where this was going. Emma looked animated and determined to make her point.

"Love him for who he is, Sophie. Find him again – the spirit that you fell in love with. He's still there. You know, you can still find him in that way. You're lucky. I lost the spirit that I loved. He disappeared after he and my dad had a terrible accident together."

Sophie looked at Emma and turned sheet-white. "What did you say, Emma?"

"I lost the man I loved, Sophie. He didn't only lose his leg. He lost his life. And after that, try as I could, I couldn't find him, even though I know he is still around somewhere, some place, as a spirit – or who knows, maybe he has a new body now. I can only guess. I don't know that. I had to let go and my mom and I decided to move to a new place, to try and forget the memories."

"Oh, my word, Emma, I am so, so, sorry. I had no idea that you had to go through something like that. What happened to him and your dad?" Sophie looked at Emma and realized that this was probably what had made Emma so strong, having to survive something so rough and then keep going with life. Her respect for Emma grew even more as she listened on.

"Dan was the man of my dreams. He was everything I could have wished for, and I was really lucky to have a boyfriend that Mom and Dad loved too. Everything seemed perfect. But the dreams were about to turn into a nightmare.

Dad and Dan used to do 'guy' stuff together. They went on a fishing trip not far from home – near the dam on the outskirts of our town. Like what happened to Robert, it was just one of those really bad things that life can sometimes deal out. You can't blame anyone and you can't go back and change it. It happened.

It was a freak accident. They planned to camp out near the dam for the weekend. A storm started to come up out of nowhere and they were trying to pitch their two-man tent before the rain started pouring down – they must have been eager to get it up so that they could have their shelter for the night. The experts said that a sudden flash of lightening streaked through the sky right at the inception of the storm. That was followed by ground-current arcs that reached out underneath their bodies from a massive tree trunk quite a distance away. They weren't reckless or anything and had not tried to pitch a tent near any trees. I had no idea that could happen. It was just a freak accident. No-one expected it. They had been working closely together to put up the tent and were both struck with a huge electrical force and died instantly. Their hearts just stopped.

I don't want to think about it or talk about it anymore. But I thought you should know so that I can help you and Robert. So, don't feel so sorry for yourself, Sophie, that Robert lost half a leg. You should love him and cherish him because he's still Robert. He's still the same guy. And he's still here."

"Emma, I don't know what to say. If only I'd known about this all those times I was so nasty and spiteful to you." Sophie put her arm around Emma and held her, trying to ease her own and Emma's pain. She realized in that moment, that although life was not always fair, and she had been dealt a bitter blow, she could and should still be true to her Robert and work things out with him. This beautiful Emma from her little town up in the province of

Mpumalanga (which meant "the place where the sun rises" in the local language), had brought sunshine and wisdom to her and their group of friends. She held Emma close as Emma shed the first few tears she'd allowed to flow since arriving in her new home.

Chapter 10

It was a hot late afternoon in Ocean Sound and the only respite if you didn't have aircon, was to cool off in the sea or in a swimming pool if you had one. Today, the friends were all hanging out at Robert's house. His sister, Cindy was up from Cape Town for a short holiday. She and Jenna were firm friends and everyone was having a great time in the cool water of Robert's swimming pool at his parents' house.

Robert and Sophie were back together now and their relationship was stronger than ever. They both knew that they had one person to thank for that. Ever since Emma had told her full story to Sophie, she came to her senses and realized how much she had to be grateful for and appreciate in her life. It had been a real wake-up call.

Robert was delighted, because, as he had told Emma when they met to try out his diving, he had never, ever stopped loving his Sophie. Both Robert and Sophie now knew that nothing could ever come between them. They had survived this test and worked things out. He forgave Sophie for her rejection of him as he knew that deep down, she was hurting herself more than she hurt him. She just needed some guidance, which Emma provided in the most caring and helpful way.

Emma was due to arrive a little later as she had to work late at the bank at month-end. She would meet Robert's sister tonight and was excited to get there as soon as she could. Meantime, her friends had already started the pool party and were having a good time together.

Mark was feeling a bit left out with Jenna and Cindy renewing their friendship and catching up on things – usually he hung out with Jenna and that way he escaped the pressure to hook up with a girl. He was quite a shy guy, and felt that at the right time, the right girl would come into his life. If not, then so be it. He could just as easily remain a bachelor – or so he'd thought until Emma had arrived on the scene.

~~~

"Rob, you have to help me out, man," said Mark, nervously turning his glass of soda round and round in his huge hand. He had called Robert aside to talk to him at the plastic table set under the tree, a little distance from where the others were swimming in the pool. "I thought you were going to fall for Emma, so I kept out of that when Sophie was giving you the run-around. But now that you've got your girl back, I have to tell you, Rob, I really, really like Emma. You know – really – not just as a friend. I think the love-thing has finally come to bite me Rob - and I need some coaching from the expert around here. I don't know what to do. Every time I approach her, she's so super friendly but she holds me off. She doesn't let it go any further. She's such a sweet girl, I don't know how to deal with it. Am I that off-putting to the girls?"

"Mark, don't be an idiot! You're a catch, man! You could make many girls happy. You just need the right one. The girl who lands you is a very lucky person!" grinned Robert, delighted that he could finally help his friend Mark, to get together with someone as nice as Emma.

"She has a history, Mark. It's not what you think. It's something I don't really want to discuss right now as she told Sophie in confidence. But if there's anyone around here who deserves a lucky break, it's definitely our sweet Emma!"

Robert suddenly had an idea. "Mark, leave it to me. If you want to get closer to Emma, I have a plan."

The rest of the afternoon and evening was spent frolicking in the pool, playing ball games and ending with a delicious barbecue on the grill that Rob had set up near the table. Sophie, Jenna and Cindy had prepared some delicious salads and everyone had a great time.

Emma had arrived to a happy group cooling off and chatting around the pool and despite her late arrival, quickly felt at home at the party. She was introduced to Cindy and took to her immediately. She was quite similar in personality to Robert and they found they had a lot in common in terms of their work, as Cindy worked for a financial institution in Cape Town. She too, had moved away from her home town and had to start anew with strangers in a new place. So, they understood each other well.

After an afternoon of swimming, burning in the hot, December sun until the evening breeze brought some mild relief, and eating ravenously once the food came off the grill; everyone was happy to help tidy up and start making their way home.

"Bye guys! Thanks for a lovely time!" said Emma enthusiastically, as she left first, to clear the way for the other cars that had parked prior to her arrival. "See you all at the next game on Saturday!"

"She's great, isn't she?" said Robert to Cindy, as Emma drove off waving cheerily. "We think that she and Mark would make a good pair. We're on it!" He smiled a little sneakily at his sister. Cindy agreed. She knew that once Robert set his mind on something he usually got what he wanted. But this was a question of love – that would also have to be up to Mark and Emma. In fact, it was only up to them and what they wanted.

"Wish you luck, Rob, it would be a good match." She smiled and went off to chat with Sophie, who was having some tea in the shade of the huge avocado pear tree a little distance from the pool.

Chapter 11

"Emma, we need to have a talk," said Sophie to her friend. They were doing their usual Saturday morning visit at Emma's apartment. "And this time I'm bringing Robert along."

"What's up, Sophie? I thought everything was going great with you and Robert now," said Emma with a concerned look.

"Thanks to you, Em, it's never been better. Honestly, Robert and I owe you so much. You said exactly the right things to me to make me wake up and smell the coffee. And boy, does Robert make great coffee by the way! No – this is about something else, Emma. We'll see you at Robert's cottage later. Let's make it 3 p.m."

Emma arrived at Robert's parents' house 5 minutes before 3. She tooted her car hooter for Robert to know she had arrived. Within a few seconds, the remote-controlled automatic gate started sliding open so that Emma could park her mom's car inside the property.

They were still sharing a car as they worked close to each other in the town and Emma was saving for her own little run-around when she could afford to pay for it in cash. Luckily, Mom liked to relax at home mostly when she wasn't busy at work and she didn't need to go anywhere that afternoon.

"Hi Emma!" said Martha, Robert's mom, as she came out the front door to ensure Emma had enough space to park. "Robert and Sophie are round the back in his cottage. You're welcome to take the short cut through the house."

Martha, like everyone else, had grown very fond of Emma and was really happy that she and her mom had moved to their town. Martha and John both knew that Emma had something to do with Robert and Sophie finding peace again in their relationship. And they were very grateful for that.

"Thanks, Martha," said Emma, giving her a hug in greeting before traipsing down the hallway towards the back door just outside the kitchen. She made her way down the path past the typically dark-green, large-leafed bushes of the KwaZulu-Natal South Coast and saw Robert coming out to greet her, with Sophie close behind him.

"Hi Em!" Robert and Sophie hugged her warmly and invited her into Robert's 1-bedroom cottage that he'd occupied in his parents' garden from when he was still in high school. While Robert was studying and working, the arrangement was that he'd stay on in his parents' garden cottage for a small rental so that he could save a good deposit for a nice home of his own once he completed his studies and found his own place to settle.

His little home was quite spacious for a garden cottage. Emma sat down in a comfortable chair near the window where the ocean breeze wafted into the space, fluttering the curtains that Sophie had lovingly made for Robert when he first moved in here.

"Tea or juice?" asked Sophie from the kitchen area.

"I'd love some of that delicious home-made mango juice that you gave me last time – if you have some from your garden mangoes," said Emma happily. She liked this space, and it was so nice to see Robert and Sophie so comfortably together.

"Coming right up!" said Sophie, bringing through a drink for everyone.

"OK guys, what's up that I got this special invite?" asked Emma, not able to contain her curiosity any longer.

"Emma, you helped us more than words or deeds can ever thank you," said Robert. You had such wisdom and insight when Sophie was going through a really rough time after my accident in the ocean. We are so happy together now, and we've never looked back since that day that you talked to her."

"I'm happy for you guys," said Emma, her brown eyes glistening with emotion.

"Emma, I know that it wasn't easy for you to open up to me about your own tragic circumstances that led to you and your mom coming down here. I know you only mentioned that to give me a wake-up call," said Sophie.

Emma dropped her head a little, not liking where this conversation was going. But she didn't want to get too annoyed with her friends.

"I didn't want to bring it up and hurt you and make you feel that pain again, Emma, but since you helped me to move on from my pain, Rob and I really want to help you to move on from yours."

Emma looked up at her friends, with tears in her eyes now. "You guys are the only ones in the town that know from me what occurred. I hope you don't mention it to anyone else, please. I hate to have anyone remind me of it or make me think about this."

"I know, Emma," said Sophie softly, "I'm sorry we need to mention it now to you – we haven't told anyone else, I promise. But the point is, we *do* know about it and we know that that might make things tricky when a guy reaches out to you, Em."

"No-one can ever replace Dan," said Emma so quietly, she could scarcely be heard above the sea breeze gently blowing into the room.

"We know that, Emma, and we understand." Sophie put her hand on

Emma's and wondered if she and Robert were doing the right thing. She could feel Emma's grief and trapped pain and felt desperately sad for her. But she drew in a deep breath and decided that the right thing to do was exactly what Emma had done for her. They needed to help Emma to leave the past behind and move into the future, with all of the love that she had in her. She didn't need to stifle that love because of her loss.

"Emma, when you helped me, it also wasn't easy. I thought that the "easy" way out was to not confront what was actually happening with me and Robert. I thought the "easy" way to move on was to ignore it and pretend everything was fine without Robert. It wasn't the "easy" way out, Em, and you knew that. You knew that you had to shock me into seeing what I was doing to myself and to Robert. You were courageous enough to put my nose into it and get me to look at my life and where I was going by not facing up to things. Sometimes I hated you for doing that, but in the end, I loved you for bringing Robert and me back together."

It was now Emma's turn to listen to her own wisdom coming back at her. She understood that there was no point now in resisting this communication or protesting. Her friends were genuine about helping her. Difficult as it was for Emma, she gave Sophie and Robert her full attention.

"Emma, there is someone in this town who is hopelessly in love with you," said Robert softly, after Sophie had set the scene for Emma to be willing to listen to them. "He doesn't know your history, Emma, we didn't say a word. And he's shy enough as it is, so it's really going to take two of you to make this happen. He confided in me that he wants to get to know you better, but, being the kind of guy that he is, he's not going to push it past a good point if it's not right for you."

Emma felt her heart start to beat faster and faster. She had not expected something like this when she so cheerfully tooted outside the gate to be let in. She felt trapped, highly emotional and quite out of control. The mixed emotions flooding through her made her face go red, then pale, then red again. She was totally flustered and speechless. She tried to take a sip of the delicious mango juice that Sophie had brought her, but the glass clattered noisily on the table as her hand shook uncontrollably.

"Listen guys, no-one can ever replace Dan," she finally managed to whisper again.

"Rob, please give us a moment," said Sophie, motioning for Robert to leave and go outside into the garden. Sophie had never seen her new-found friend in such a state. She was starting to worry about her and knew she had to calm Emma down.

"Here, Em," she said kindly, holding up the glass for Emma to take a sip of the cold mango juice. Sophie knew that the sugar from the sweet mango would help a bit. Again, she wondered if she and Robert had made the right decision to raise this with Emma. She didn't like to see her friend suffering like this. Then she thought of herself and how she'd had to overcome doubts before she could move on.

"Emma, if Dan were here right now, what would he want for you?" she suddenly asked. "Would he want you to continue to live a life without a special someone at your side, staying more or less isolated from ever entering into a proper relationship again?"

Emma listened. She was feeling a little less shaky now, and took the glass from Sophie and drank a bit more juice.

What would Dan want? She thought about the question Sophie had posed. She didn't know the answer. Dan wasn't here anymore, so how could she know. Emma knew that the night she lost her dad and Dan in one flash, that she had to be strong for her mom, because that's all that she had left of her family. From that moment, Emma had stifled all her sorrow and grief. She'd covered it up in her mind and put a protective shield around it and vowed never to think about it again. The problem was, the more she covered it up, the more it haunted her every awake moment; and often, the horror of that incident entered into her nightmares as well. This was the first time someone who really cared about her was asking her to consider these things.

She and Mom had talked it over, but Emma never let go with her mom, for fear of bringing all the pain back for Mom. She too, had lost the man she loved – for a lot longer than Emma and Dan had been together. So they always skirted around the thing and were never truly honest with each other about their feelings.

Now, here was Sophie, the girl who had once called her a "bitch", sitting quietly with her and asking her to take a look at her past and move into the present and future.

"Sophie," Emma's voice quivered as she tried to talk, "I'm going to need to cry a bit, I think. I never cried about this. I bottled it all up. I think I would like to walk in the garden with you if you don't mind."

The tears were already streaming down Emma's face as she struggled to get her words out. Sophie gently took her by the arm and took her outside.

She motioned to Robert, who was near the back door of his parents' house to leave them alone for a bit and to go inside the main house. Sophie knew where Emma wanted to go. There was a section of the garden that had several massive avocado pear trees and mango trees. The house was built on a piece of land that used to be a fruit farm and the trees had remained, bearing delicious seasonal fruits every year. The trees also provided a bit of a hideaway and once you had entered past the biggest of the trees, no-one would even know you were in there.

"Thanks, Sophie, just walk with me, please," Emma sobbed. And sobbed and sobbed and sobbed. She let out all the pent-up emotion that she'd lived with since that dreaded day when her life had been torn apart. She stopped thinking about anything and just cried her heart out. Now it was Sophie providing the Kleenex. She knew that she didn't need to say anything to Emma, but to just let Emma have this relief by unleashing the built-up sorrow.

Eventually, the grief abated a little and the two girls sat on the old, rusty bench near the pawpaw tree.

"Thanks, Sophie, for being there for me," said Emma, her eyes red and swollen.

"You were there for me, Emma, it's the least I can do."

"Sophie, I think I know who it is, who has fallen in love with me. I just couldn't handle it when he tried to reach. I didn't feel good, pushing him away and pretending I wasn't interested. He's such a nice guy. I hate to hurt someone, but I just couldn't help myself.

"It's OK, Emma. I'm sure he'll understand once you get to know each other better as a couple. Are you willing to give it a try? Nothing would make us all happier than if you and Mark got together."

Emma smiled. She was right. She knew it was Mark. She drew in a deep breath and looked at the tall trees all around them. It felt so peaceful and cool out here. This was a good place to make decisions for the future.

"OK Sophie, let me try this one step at a time," said Emma, managing at last to smile, despite her puffy eyes and wet face.

The girls went back to Robert's cottage and Emma washed her face and tidied herself up. Robert had landed up visiting with his parents inside the house. He knew the girls had to do what they needed to do and left them to it. Emma finished drinking her mango juice and said it would be OK for Sophie to call Robert back to his cottage.

As Robert walked cheerfully down the path, Sophie heard his mobile phone ringing in the cottage. Before Robert could get there, she picked it up to see who was calling.

With a twinkle in her eye, she turned to Emma, who had totally regained her composure by now. "It's Mark calling, Emma. Who is going to take this call? You or me?"

Emma started giggling. "You're a real treat, Sophie! Just give that phone to Robert!" as Robert entered the cottage.

Epilogue

It was three months since Mark and Emma had started dating. The town now had two glamour couples. Everyone was so happy for Emma and Mark. They seemed to be made for each other. Emma had finally found the answer to the question that Sophie had asked her. She knew with all her heart, that Dan would have wanted her to love again and not waste all the love that was inside her, on a lonely existence with nobody to share it with at her side.

Susan adored her daughter's new boyfriend and the happiness of Emma helped her to overcome her past loss, too.

"Hey guys, you're all invited to the provincial diving championships next week in Durban. Yours truly is competing," said Robert happily as they met on their Saturday morning promenade walk. These days, Susan, Martha and John joined the youngsters in their walk. The town had healed after the shark attack. The nets and drumlines were regularly serviced by the Sharks Board; swimmers were safe on the beaches and in the sea and everyone had learned from the accident and moved on. Ocean Sound was a happy, thriving town again. Emma and Susan never looked back. And Emma and Mark, Sophie and Robert only looked forward to a happy future.

The End

If you enjoyed "A Love Story at the Seaside", you will love my novel "A Love Story from the Heart". You can find this and other stories and audio books on my Amazon Author Page.

About the Author

Any reader can find entertainment and a sweet and clean romance in each of Terry's books, but beyond the entertainment, there is always a special message which is enlightening and which makes us feel better about the world around us and our relationships.

Terry helps us to see the brightness of the world and reminds us of how easy it is to put back values of kindness and care in any relationship.

Once you've found what's between the pages of a Terry Atkinson romance, you'll see why readers also say that they will read these stories more than once.

Although Terry has lived, studied and worked in Canada, the USA, the UK and Australia, she has been happily married to her husband, Dave, for twenty-five years and they live in their beloved South Africa.

Terry's sweet romances always contain useful tips to keep your relationships happy. Many of her books are set in her home country, but equally, she rights for couples everywhere.

Contact:

terry@terryatkinsonbooks.com

or

terryatkinsonauthor@gmail.com

Author Page:

terryatkinsonbooks.com

More Books by the Author

For a selection of further books, please see Terry's Author Page on Amazon.

https://www.amazon.com/Terry-Atkinson/e/B00HBR5L0O

Happy Reading!

www.ingramcontent.com/pod-product-compliance
Lightning Source LLC
Chambersburg PA
CBHW030714220526
45463CB00005B/2045